Table of Contents

Pre & Post Assessment...page 4

Food Diary..page 5

Step Tracker...page 6

Water Tracker..page 7

Rationale & Goal..page 8

Knowing Your Numbers..page 10

Get Ready, Set, Move...page 15

Back To The Basics..page 19

Sugar High...page 27

I Need A Break!..page 30

Getting Your Protein In..page 33

S.T.o.M.P...page 38

Portion Size/Serving Size Examples.......................page 43

The Lifeswitch Plan

"Making that switch, live an abundant life!"

Your Name:_____

Date:_____

Variables	Pre-Assessment	Post-Assessment
DATE		
Height		
Weight		
Body Mass Index		
Blood Pressure		
Glucose		
Total Cholesterol		
LDL-Cholesterol		
HDL-Cholesterol		
Triglycerides		

Food Diary

	Breakfast	Snack	Lunch	Snack	Dinner
Sun.					
Mon.					
Tues.					
Wed.					
Thurs.					
Fri.					
Sat.					

STEP TRACKER

Weeks	Week 1	Week 2	Week 3	Week 4	Week 5	Week 6	Week 7	Week 8
EXAMPLE	7000	7500	9000	10000	12500	15000	14750	15000
SUN								
MON								
TUES								
WED								
THURS								
FRI								
SAT								
Total								

WATER TRACKER

Weeks	Week 1	Week 2	Week 3	Week 4	Week 5	Week 6	Week 7	Week 8
EXAMPLE	24 oz	30 oz	54 oz	58 oz	60 oz	64 oz	64 oz	64 oz
SUN								
MON								
TUES								
WED								
THURS								
FRI								
SAT								
Total								

Your Rationale & Goal

I joined the Lifeswitch Plan because:

_____

_____

By changing my lifestyle (healthy eating and being active), it will help me to:

_____

_____

> **The Lifeswitch Plan is designed to help you reach a healthy balance.**
>
> **The goals for this plan are to:**
>
> **1. Lose weight through healthy eating.**
>
> **2. Engage in physical activity.**
>
> **By making these changes in your lifestyle, over time will help to reverse the effects of chronic disease.**

The Lifeswitch Plan will help you:

A. Learn the facts about healthy eating.

B. Learn the facts about engaging in physical activity

C. Learn what makes it hard to eat healthy and be active.

D. Learn about vegetarianism and how it can improve your health.

The Goals of Lifeswitch Will Be to Help You:

1. Lose 7% of your weight through making healthy choices.

Your goal will be to weigh _____ pounds or less.

2. Accumulate 10,000 steps/day

OR

Do 2 ½ hours of brisk, physical activity each week.

(Example: Take a brisk walk for 30 minutes 5 days/week)

**This plan is a gradual progression of incorporating lifestyle change.

Reaching the Goals of Lifeswitch will help you to:

1. Control and even reverse type-2 diabetes.

> Researchers investigated whether consuming a low-fat, vegetarian diet alters glycemic and lipid levels. Results showed that the low-fat vegetarian diet was associated with significant reductions in fasting serum glucose concentration and body weight (Nicholson, et al., 1999).

2. Look and feel better.

> A survey by Norwegian researchers found that those who engaged in any exercise, even a small amount, reported improved mental health compared with Norwegians who, despite the tempting nearness of mountains and fjords, never got out and exercised.

During the first week, the focus is to get a better understanding of the definitions that can help us understand cholesterol, blood pressure, body mass index. These health parameters help us to understand how our body works and provides us with an understanding of our risk. On page 4 you should have seen a blank table. This table will give you an opportunity to jot down your numbers.

During session #1 you will obtain a crash course on various topics and how it relates to your health and wellness.

Cholesterol

Cholesterol is a fat (lipid) which is produced by the liver and is crucial for normal body functioning. Cholesterol exists in the outer layer of every cell in our body and has many functions.

Its functions are to:

- It builds and maintains cell membranes (outer layer), it prevents crystallization of hydrocarbons in the membrane
- It is essential for determining which molecules can pass into the cell and which cannot (cell membrane permeability)
- It is involved in the production of sex hormones (androgens and estrogens)
- It is essential for the production of hormones released by the adrenal glands (cortisol, corticosterone, aldosterone, and others)
- It aids in the production of bile
- It converts sunshine to vitamin D
- It is important for the metabolism of fat soluble vitamins, including vitamins A, D, E, and K
- It insulates nerve fibers

Cholesterol is carried in the blood by molecules called lipoproteins. A lipoprotein is any complex or compound containing both lipid (fat) and protein. Four numbers you should be aware of are:

- **LDL (low density lipoprotein)** - people often refer to it as *bad cholesterol*. LDL carries cholesterol from the liver to cells. If too much is carried, too much for the cells to use, there can be a harmful buildup of LDL. This lipoprotein can increase the risk of arterial disease if levels rise too high. Most human blood contains approximately 70% LDL - this may vary, depending on the person.
- **HDL (high density lipoprotein)** - people often refer to it as *good cholesterol*. Experts say HDL prevents arterial disease. HDL does the opposite of LDL - HDL takes the cholesterol away from the cells and back to the liver. In the liver it is either broken down or expelled from the body as waste.
- **Triglycerides** - these are the chemical forms in which most fat exists in the body, as well as in food. They are present in blood plasma. Triglycerides, in association with cholesterol, form the plasma lipids (blood fat). Triglycerides in plasma originate either from fats in our food, or are made in the body from other energy sources, such as carbohydrates. Calories we consume but are not used immediately by our tissues are converted into triglycerides and stored in fat cells. When your body needs energy and there is no food as an energy source, triglycerides will be released from fat cells and used as energy.
- **Total Cholesterol** - is a measure of LDL cholesterol, HDL cholesterol, and other lipid components. Doctors recommend total cholesterol levels below 200.

LDL-Cholesterol	
Desirable	<200 mg/dL
Borderline high	200-239 mg/dL
High	240 mg/dL

HDL-Cholesterol	
60 and above	High; Optimal
Less than: 40 in men 50 in women	Low; Risk factor for HD

Triglycerides	
Normal	<150
Mildly High	150-199
High	200-499
Very High	500 or higher

Total Cholesterol	
Desirable	<200
Mildly High	200-239
High	240 and above

Blood Pressure

Classification	Systolic Blood Pressure		Diastolic Blood Pressure
Low	<90	OR	<60
Normal	<120	OR	<80
Prehypertension	120-139	OR	80-89
High: Stage 1 HTN	140-159	OR	90-99
High: Stage 2 HTN	≥160	OR	≥100

Body Mass Index - Body Mass Index (BMI) is a number calculated from a person's weight and height. BMI provides a reliable indicator of body fatness for most people and is used to screen for weight categories that may lead to health problems.

Underweight	<18.5
Normal Weight	18.5-24.9
Overweight	25-29.9
Obesity	>30

Glucose- A blood glucose test measures the amount of a type of sugar, called glucose, in your blood. Glucose comes from carbohydrate foods. Carbohydrates are the main source of energy used by the body.

There are several different types of blood glucose tests that are used:

A. Fasting blood sugar- this test measures blood glucose after you have not eaten for at least 8 hours. This test is often done to check for prediabetes and diabetes.

B. Random blood sugar- measures blood glucose regardless of when you last ate.

C. Oral glucose tolerance test -is used to diagnose prediabetes and diabetes.

Lifeswitch Action Plan for the week

STEPS/GOAL 1: Creating a food diary!

Refer to page 4 to jot down everything you eat for the week, everything.

Question 1: How do you **plan** to achieve your goal?

_____

_____

Question 2: How **confident** are you that you can achieve your goal?

How CONFIDENT are you that you will succeed with your plan? (0=not confident; 10=Confident)
0   1   2   3   4   5   6   7   8   9   10

Question 3: Are there any **obstacles** that may hinder you from achieving your goal?

_____

_____

Question 4. What **strategies** are you going to put in place to help you achieve your goal?

_____

_____

The focus for this week is to start getting active daily. Most of us walk throughout the day. We can use that form of physical activity to jump start our calorie burning and start moving.

Exercise has always been a lifestyle tool that helps keep the body strong and healthy.

Studies have shown that exercise:

1. Reduces anxiety

Researchers at the University of Missouri-Columbia showed that a relatively high-intensity exercise is superior in reducing stress and anxiety that may lead to heart disease. Moreover, the researchers found that high-intensity exercise especially benefits women.

2. Reduces blood sugar

After analyzing the results of 47 randomized clinical trials, the researchers also found that exercising for longer periods of time was better at bringing blood sugar levels down than exercising more intensively (Schaan, et al. 2011).

3. Reduces blood pressure

Regular aerobic exercise decreased systolic blood pressure by 3.84 mm Hg and diastolic blood pressure by 2.58 mm Hg in people who were previously inactive. Exercise lowered blood pressure in all groups of people, including those who had hypertension or normal blood pressure; were obese or of normal weight; and was black, white, or Asian (Whelton et. al., 2002).

4. Increases high-density lipoproteins

Dr Satoru Kodama (Ochanomizu University, Tokyo, Japan) and colleagues showed that the effect of aerobic training resulted in a 2.53-mg/dL increase in HDL-cholesterol levels. With each 1-mg/dL increment in HDL-cholesterol levels associated with a 2% to 3% decreased risk of cardiovascular disease (Kodama S et al. *Arch Intern Med* 2007; 167:999-1008).

Therefore the goal for this week is to:

1. Track your steps daily for the week with your pedometer (you can download a free app to help you track your steps)

Ways to Increase Your Steps
- Park at the outer edges of parking lots instead of as close as possible to stores, health clubs, church, etc.
- Get up and walk during television commercials.
- Pace while you have phone conversations. In a five-minute conversation you can add about 100 steps.
- Take stairs instead of elevators or escalators.
- Walk and talk with friends and family instead of sitting and talking.
- Use part of every break or lunch time to add a few steps to your day.

Water

Water is a must have in order to live a healthy lifestyle. Water makes up for 70% of our body weight. We can live with food for a period of time, but we can only live without water for a couple of days. Water does a couple of things to keep our body working effectively:

Benefits of Water

- **Water serves as a lubricant**

- **Water forms the fluid that surround joints**

- **Water regulates the body temperature**

- **Water helps to regulate metabolism**

- **Water can help to decrease the risk of colon cancer**

Your second goal for this week is to:

2. Track your water consumption.

Lifeswitch Action Plan for the week

STEPS/GOAL 1: Track your daily steps this week!

Question 1: How do you **plan** to achieve your track your water intake?

_____

_____

Question 2: How **confident** are you that you can achieve your goal?

How CONFIDENT are you that you will succeed with your plan? (0=not confident; 10=Confident)
0   1   2   3   4   5   6   7   8   9   10

Question 3: Are there any **obstacles** that may hinder you from achieving your goal?

_____

_____

4. What **strategies** are you going to put in place to help you achieve your goal?

_____

_____

Lifeswitch Action Plan for the week

WATER/GOAL 2: Track water consumption this week!

Question 1: How do you **plan** to achieve your water goal?

_____

_____

Question 2: How **confident** are you that you can achieve your goal?

How CONFIDENT are you that you will succeed with your plan? (0=not confident; 10=Confident)
0   1   2   3   4   5   6   7   8   9   10

Question 3: What **obstacles** that may hinder you from achieving your goal?

_____

_____

Question 4: What **strategies** are you going to put in place to help you achieve your goal?

_____

_____

Fruits & Vegetables

The focus for this week is to go "back to the basics" and increase your fruits and vegetables. For most of us growing up, we had a regular intake of fruits and vegetables. However as we got older, other foods have been ingested that took the place of these healthy choices. We would like to use this time to focus on the benefits of incorporating fruits and vegetables in our diet.

Studies have shown that:

1. Vegetables and type 2 diabetes

> Researchers investigated fruit and vegetable intake and incidence of type 2 diabetes and found that increasing daily intake of green leafy vegetables could significantly reduce the risk of type 2 diabetes (BMJ. 2010, 341:c4229)

2. Vegetables, fruit and disease

> The higher the average daily intake of fruits and vegetables, the lower the chances of developing cardiovascular disease. Compared with those in the lowest category of fruit and vegetable intake (less than 1.5 servings a day), those who averaged 8 or more servings a day were 30 percent less likely to have had a heart attack or stroke (JNatl Cancer Inst, 2004.96(21):p.1577-84)

3. Vegetables and cardiovascular disease

> Researchers combined findings from multiple studies and examined coronary heart disease and stroke separately and found a similar protective effect: Individuals who ate more than 5 servings of fruits and vegetables per had roughly a 20 percent lower risk of coronary heart disease and stroke, compared with individuals who ate less than 3 servings per day (J Hum Hypertens, 2007. 21(9): p. 717-28., Fruit and vegetable consumption and stroke: meta-analysis of cohort studies. Lancet, 2006. 367(9507): p. 320-6.

4. Fruit and vegetable intake and incidence of type 2 diabetes

In a study of over 66,000 women in the Nurses' Health Study, 85,104 women from the Nurses' Health Study II, and 36,173 men from the Health Professionals Follow-up Study who were free of major chronic diseases, findings suggested that greater consumption of whole fruits – especially blueberries, grapes, and apples – is associated with a lower risk of type 2 diabetes.

Therefore the goals for this week are to:

1. Consume 2 servings of fruits/day

2. Consume 3 servings of vegetables/day

5-a-Day Fruit & Vegetable List
(All fruits help to reduce the risk of some cancers)

Blue Fruits & Vegetables These fruits and vegetables improve memory and aging.

FRUITS

Blackberries

Blueberries

Black Currants

Black Olives

Dried Plums

Elderberries

Purple Figs

Purple Grapes

Plums

Raisins

VEGETABLES

Purple Asparagus

Purple Cabbage

Purple Carrots

Eggplant

Purple Belgian Endive

Purple Peppers

Potatoes (Purple Fleshed

Black Salsify

Yellow/Orange Fruits & Vegetables These fruits and vegetables improve heart health, vision and your immune system.

FRUITS

Yellow Apples

Apricots

Cape Gooseberries

Cantaloupe

Carambola (Starfruit)

Yellow Figs

Grapefruit

Golden KiwiFruit

Lemons

Mangoes

Nectarines

Oranges

Papayas

Peaches

Yellow Pears

Persimmons

Pineapples

Tangerines

Yellow Watermelon

VEGETABLES

Yellow Beets

Butternut Squash

Carrots

Yellow Peppers

Yellow Potatoes

Pumpkin

Yellow Summer Squash

Sweet corn

Yellow Tomatoes

Red Fruits & Vegetables

These fruits and vegetables improve memory and heart health

FRUITS

Red Apples

Blood Oranges

Cherries

Cranberries

Red Grapes

Pink/Red Grapefruit

Red Pears

Pomegranates

Raspberries

Strawberries

Watermelon

VEGETABLES

Beets

Red Peppers

Radishes

Radicchio

Red Onions

Red Potatoes

Rhubard

Tomatoes

White Fruits & Vegetables (These fruits and vegetables improve heart health and cholesterol levels.

FRUITS

Bananas

Cherimoyas

Dates

White Nectarines

White Peaches

Brown Pears

VEGETABLES

Cauliflower

Garlic

Ginger

Jerusalem Artichokes

Jicama

Kohlrabi

Mushrooms

Onions

Parsnips

Potatoes (White Fleshed)

Shallots

Turnips

White Corn

Green Fruits & Vegetables These fruits help improve vision, bones and teeth.

FRUITS

Avocadoes

Green Apples

Green Grapes

Green Olives

Honeydew

Kiwifruit

Limes

Green Pears

VEGETABLES

Artichokes

Arugula

Asparagus

Broccoflower

Broccoli

Broccoli Rabe

Brussels Sprouts

Chinese Cabbage

Celery

Chayote Squash

Cucumbers

Endive

Leafy Greens

Lettuce

Leeks

Green Onions

Okra

Fresh Pas

Green Peppers

Snow Peas

Spinach

Sugar Snap Peas

Watercress

Fiber

Fiber refers to carbohydrates that cannot be digested. Fiber can be found in all plants that are eaten for food, that including fruits, vegetables, grains, and legumes. Not all fibers are the same. Fibers from grains are referred to as cereal fiber. There are soluble fibers that partially dissolve in water. And there are insoluble fiber does not dissolve in water.

Benefits of Fiber

- Helps lower cholesterol

- Helps with constipation

- When combined with CHOs it slows absorption of sugars and regulates insulin response

- Makes us feel full, discouraging overeating

Sources of Fiber (examples)

- Whole-grain breads and cereals

- Fruits and vegetables

- Legumes and almonds

Current Recommendations/Daily Goal:

Gender	Fiber Intake (grams)
Male	30-38
Female	21-25

There are two types of fiber:

	Insoluble Fiber	Soluble Fiber
Functions	• Move bulk through the intestines • Control and balance the pH (acidity) in the intestines	• Bind with fatty acids • **Prolong stomach emptying** time so that sugar is released and absorbed more slowly
Benefits	• Promote regular bowel movement and **prevent constipation** • Remove toxic waste through colon in less time • Help prevent colon cancer by keeping an optimal pH in intestines to prevent microbes from producing cancerous substances	• Power total cholesterol and LDLs therefore reducing the risk of heart disease • **Regulate blood sugar** for people with diabetes
Sources	• Vegetables such as green beans and dark green leafy vegetables • Fruit skins and root vegetable skins • Whole-wheat products • Wheat bran • Corn bran • Seeds & Nuts	• Oat/Oat bran • Dried beans and peas • Nuts • Barley • Flax seed • Fruits such as oranges and apples • Vegetables such as carrots • Psyllium husk

Studies have shown that incorporating more fiber in our diet:

1. The effect of fiber and high blood pressure

> Researchers evaluated the results of 25 studies on the effects on blood pressure of adding fiber to the diet. The type of fiber added to the diet in the studies included fruit, cereal, fiber pills, and vegetables. The results showed that adding fiber to the diet was associated with a significant reduction in both systolic and diastolic blood pressure in people with high blood pressure (Whelton, et al., 2005)

2. Helps to lower blood glucose levels

> Psyllium seed, derived from a type of Mediterranean plaintain, contains high quantities of soluble and insoluble fiber that improve glucose levels In the meta-study -- a review of previously published research -- 10.2 g of psyllium per day along with a low sugar diet decreased HbA1c -- a reflection of glucose levels over several months preceding the test -- and glucose levels after meals both decreased (Barjorek & Morello. *Annals of Pharmacotherapy*, 2010; 44(11):1786-92)

3. Helps with weight loss

> A review summarizing the effects of high- versus low-fiber diet interventions found that the high-fiber diets in 20 of 22 studies resulted in weight loss. Using pooled data from 12 of the intervention studies that did not control energy intake, the authors found that the participants on the higher-fiber diets lost significantly more weight than those on the lower-fiber diets (Howarth et al., 2001; American Journal of Clinical Nutrition, 73:1010-1018).

Lifeswitch Action Plan for the week

F/V GOAL 3: Use the food diary by plugging in your 2 servings of fruits and 3+ serving of vegetables/day this week.

Question 1: How do you **plan** to achieve your fruit/vegetable goal?

Now is a good time to use your food diary. The food diary is going to help you create your personalized meal plan. You may be already consuming fruits and vegetables, the plan is to make it the appropriate serving size and consistent.

_____

_____

Question 2: How **confident** are you that you can achieve your goal?

How CONFIDENT are you that you will succeed with your plan? (0=not confident; 10=Confident)
0   1   2   3   4   5   6   7   8   9   10

Question 3: What **obstacles** that may hinder you from achieving your goal?

_____

_____

Question 4: What **strategies** are you going to put in place to help you achieve your goal?

_____

_____

Carbohydrates (CHOs)

Our bodies' preferred energy source is carbohydrate.

There are two forms of carbohydrate in foods:

Simple Carbohydrates (Sugar)

Added sugars (added to sodas, breakfast cereals, baked goods, frozen desserts, candies, and other sweets)

-White table sugar (100% sucrose)

-Molasses

-Brown sugar

-Honey

-High fructose corn syrup

-Concentrated fruit juice sweetener

Naturally occurring sugars

Complex Carbohydrates (starch)

Refined, processed foods (low fiber)

-"Enriched wheat flour" breads and cereals

-White rice, White pasta

-Instant potatoes and French fried potato

-Fruit sugar (fructose)

-Milk sugar (lactose)

Whole foods (high fiber)

-**"Whole" wheat or grain breads and cereals**

-**Oats, brown and wild rice, whole wheat pasta**

-**Beans, peas, whole vegetables and fruits**

CHO summary:

-All carbohydrates are broken down in the body to sugar (blood sugar or glucose). And all carbohydrates fuel our body and brain in the same way.

-Sugars (when added to foods) are a more concentrated form of CHO and calories

-Added sugars have few, if any vitamins/ minerals

-Added sugars (also refined, low fiber starchy foods) are absorbed more quickly, resulting in a rapid increase in blood sugar levels.

Take Home Point

-**A healthy eating plan consists of wholesome CHOs that include whole grains, beans, vegetables and fruits.**

Whole Grains

A whole grain consists of 4 parts:

a. **The germ**- the nutrient inner part

b. **The endosperm**- the soft white, starch inside portion

c. **The bran**- the fibrous coating around the grain

d. **The husk**- the outer inedible shell

We are all bombarded with different types of breads to buy. You may have come across terms called refined and enriched.

Refined/ refinement is the process that removes all but the endosperm portion of the grain, leaving a white, nutrient-poor, refined flour

Enrichment is the process that adds back nutrients (iron, folic acid, thiamin, niacin, riboflavin) to the white, refined flour. And all other nutrients from the whole grain (magnesium, zinc, vitamin B6, chromium, vitamin E, and fiber) are lost.

Lifeswitch Action Plan for the week

CHOs/GOAL 4: Use the food diary by plugging in your 6 healthy carbohydrate servings/day this week!

Question 1: How do you **plan** to achieve your carbohydrate goal?

The food diary is going to help you create your personalized meal plan. You may be already consuming carbohydrates, the plan is to make it the appropriate serving size, whole wheat and consistent.

_____

_____

Question 2: How **confident** are you that you can achieve your goal?

How CONFIDENT are you that you will succeed with your plan? (0=not confident; 10=Confident)
0   1   2   3   4   5   6   7   8   9   10

Question 3: What **obstacles** that may hinder you from achieving your goal?

_____

_____

Question 4: What **strategies** are you going to put in place to help you achieve your goal?

_____

_____

Stress

A specific response by the body to a stimulus, as fear or pain, that disturbs or interferes with the normal physiological equilibrium of an organism.

Eustress

Eustress is a positive form of stress, usually arises in any situation in which a person finds motivating or inspiring, examples could be engaging in sports, meeting someone famous or falling or getting married. Eustress situations are normally enjoyable and not harmful psychologically or physiologically.

Distress

Distress is the most common type of stress, having negative implications. It is defined as causing great pain, anxiety, or sorrow. Although eustress and distress can both be equally taxing on the body, and are cumulative in nature, distress puts a person in a state of extreme necessity or misfortune.

Acute Stress

An experience in response to an immediate threat that is either perceived as physical, emotional or psychological. The threat can be real or imagined. During an acute stress response, the autonomic nervous system is activated causing an increased level or cortisol, adrenalin and other hormones. These hormones cause an increase in heart rate, quickened breathing rate and higher blood pressure. Blood is shunted from the big muscles, preparing the body to fight or flight.

Chronic Stress

Chronic stress is a state of ongoing physiological arousal. This occurs when the body experiences so many stressors that the autonomic nervous system rarely has a chance to relax. This type of chronic stress response occurs all too frequently from our modern lifestyle, when issues such as a high-powered job, loneliness, busy traffic or other factors that can keep the body in a state of perceived threat.

Stress Management techniques

1. Sleep 7-8 hours a night

Getting your sleep allows your body to rejuvenate, recharge and get ready for the next day. Your body, bones and muscles need the rest.

2. Exercise regularly

Exercises help to train the body, affect the brain positively and decrease overall tension and improve self-esteem.

3. Eat healthy options daily

Healthy nutrition promotes a sense of wellbeing and encourages a greater outlook on life.

4. Manage your time

By creating tasks, goals and a list to help you with your time.

5. Take daily breaks

Daily breaks have been show to help reduce blood pressure and the monotony of life.

Lifeswitch Action Plan for the week

STRESS/GOAL 5: I plan to use _____ stress management this week!

Question 1: How do you **plan** to achieve your stress management goal?

_____

_____

Question 2: How **confident** are you that you can achieve your goal?

How CONFIDENT are you that you will succeed with your plan? (0=not confident; 10=Confident)										
0	1	2	3	4	5	6	7	8	9	10

Question 3: What **obstacles** that may hinder you from achieving your goal?

_____

_____

Question 4: What **strategies** are you going to put in place to help you achieve your goal?

_____

_____

What is Protein?

Protein is a set of molecules that are made up of different amino acids. Amino acids are combinations of carbon, hydrogen, oxygen, nitrogen and at times sulfur. Carbon, hydrogen and oxygen are the basic building blocks of many organic compounds. There are 20 different amino acids that join together to form protein. There are two types of amino acids, non-essential and essential amino acids.

Non-essential amino acids are amino acids that your body can create out of chemicals found in your body. Essential amino acids cannot be created, and therefore has to be obtained through food.

Non-essential Amino Acids

- Alanine
- Arginine
- Asparagine
- Cysteine
- Glutamic Acid
- Glutamine
- Glycine
- Proline
- Serine
- Tyrosine

Essential Amino Acids

- Histidine
- Isoleucine
- Leucine
- Lysine
- Methionine
- Phenylalanine
- Threonine
- Tryptophan
- Valine

Protein comes from animal and/or vegetable sources. Most animal sources (meat, milk, eggs, poultry, fish, and cheese) provide a "complete protein," proteins that contain all the essential amino acids. Vegetable sources (nuts, seeds, milk alternatives, grains, tofu, legumes, some vegetables and fruits) vary in obtaining the essential amino acids. However by combining a variety of foods, you can obtain adequate amounts of the needed amino acids.

Why we need protein?

Amino acids provide cells with the building material needed to grow and maintain their structure.

We need protein for:

A. Growth, maintenance and repair of cells

B. A tertiary source of energy for the body

C. The production of enzymes and hormones (ex: digestion, metabolism)

D. Help transport lipoproteins (ex: cholesterol, triglycerides)

E. The production of antibodies (immune system)

The Rationale for a Plant-based diet

We all would like to live as long as possible. And one of the things we can incorporate into our diet is proteins that are plant-based.

What does the research say?

1. Meat intake and mortality

Researchers examined relations of red, white, and processed meat intakes to risk for total and cause-specific mortality. Meat intake was estimated from a food frequency questionnaire administered at baseline. They concluded that red and processed meat intakes were associated with modest increases in total mortality, cancer mortality, and cardiovascular disease mortality (*Archives of internal medicine*, 2009; 169(6):562-571)

2. Meat vs. type 2 diabetes

Researchers examined meat consumption and risk of type 2 diabetes in a multiethnic cohort. They concluded that red and processed meat intake increase risk for diabetes irrespective of ethnicity and level of BMI (Steinbrecher et al., Meat consumption and risk of type 2 diabetes: the multiethnic cohort. (*Public health nutrition*: 14(4), 568-574).

3. Red meat consumption and mortality

Researchers examined the relationship between red meat and chronic disease by observing 37, 698 men and 83,644 women who were free of cardiovascular disease and cancer at baseline. Diet was assessed by validated food frequency questionnaires and updated every 4 years. They concluded that red meat consumption is associated with an increased risk of total, cardiovascular, and cancer mortality. Substitution of other healthy protein sources for red mead is associated with a lower mortality risk (*Journal of American medical Association*: 172(7), 555-563)

4. Vegetarian diets and new cases of type 2 diabetes

Researchers evaluated the relationship of diet to incident diabetes among non-Black and Black participants in the Adventist Health Study-2. We concluded that a vegetarian diet were associated with a substantial and independent reduction in diabetes incidence. In Blacks the dimension of the protection associated with vegetarian diets was as great as the excess risk associated with Black ethnicity (Tonstad S., Stewart K., et al. Vegetarian diets and incidence of diabetes in the Adventist Health Study-2, Nutrition Metabolism and Cardiovascular Disease, 2011).

Protein Recommendations

Gender	Age	Grams/Day
Male	19-70	56 Grams
Female	19-70	46 Grams

Retrieved on January 20, 2012, Dietary Reference Intakes report by the Institute of Medicine, 2002 from http://www.medicinenet.com/script/main/art.asp?articlekey=56691

Lifeswitch Action Plan for the week

PROTEIN/GOAL 6: Use the food diary by plugging in how many times you plan make alternative choices for my protein this week!

Question 1: How do you **plan** to achieve your protein goal?

Now is a good time to use your food diary. The food diary is going to help you create your personalized meal plan. You may be already consuming protein, the plan is to make it the chose healthier protein options, including from non-animal products, appropriate serving sizes and consistent.

_____

_____

Question 2: How **confident** are you that you can achieve your goal?

How CONFIDENT are you that you will succeed with your plan? (0=not confident; 10=Confident)
0   1   2   3   4   5   6   7   8   9   10

Question 3: What **obstacles** that may hinder you from achieving your goal?

_____

_____

Question 4: What **strategies** are you going to put in place to help you achieve your goal?

_____

_____

Why we need fats?

Fats are needed because it gives our body energy and aid in cell growth. Fats help to protect our organs, but also create some form of insulation to keep our body warm. Lastly, fats help our body to absorb some nutrients and produce hormones.

There are 4 major Fats: **saturated fats, trans fats, monounsaturated fats and polyunsaturated fats**. They are classified in two categories, bad fats and better fats.

	Saturated Fats	Trans Fats	Monounsaturated Fats	Polyunsaturated Fats
Commonly found in these foods	-Mainly from animals (beef, lamb, pork, poultry with skin, beef fat, lard, cream cheese -Some from plants (Palm, palm kernel and coconut oils	-Baked goods (pastries, biscuits, cakes, pie crusts, doughnuts and cookies)	-Vegetable oils (olive, canola, peanut and sesame -Avocadoes and olives -Nuts and seeds(almond and peanuts/peanut butter	–High in omega-6 and omega 3 (vegetable oils-soybean, corn and safflower - Nuts and seeds(almond and peanuts/peanut butter -High in Omega-3 (fatty fish)
Effect on Heart	-Raises LDL-cholesterol -Increases risk of heart disease	-Raises LDL-cholesterol -Increases risk of heart disease	-Reduces LDL-cholesterol -May lower risk of heart disease	-Reduces LDL-cholesterol -May lower risk of heart disease
Daily Limit	Less than 7% of total daily calories 2000calories 140calories/15 grams	Less than 1% of total daily calories 2000calories 20calories (2 grams)	-Total fats should be about 25%-35% of total calories	-Total fats should be about 25%-35% of total calories

Dairy

All fluid milk products and a host of foods made from milk are considered part of the dairy group. Commonly eaten dairy products consist of:

Milk (skim, 1%, 2%, whole, flavored, lactose and lactose-free)

Milk-based desserts (puddings, ice milk, frozen yogurt and ice cream)

Cheese (hard natural cheese, soft cheeses, processed cheese)

Yogurt/All yogurt (fat-free, low fat, reduced fat, whole milk yogurt)

The Rationale for Less Milk in your Diet:

1. Milk does not reduce fractures

According to the Nurses' Health Study dairy may increase risk of fractures by 50 percent.

2. Less dairy, better bones

Countries with lowest rates of dairy and calcium consumption (like those in Africa and Asia) have the lowest rates of osteoporosis.

3. Too much calcium and dairy promotes cancer

Research shows that higher intakes of both calcium and dairy products may increase a man's risk of prostate cancer by 30 to 50 percent. Dairy consumption increases the body's level insulin-like growth factor (IGF-1) -- a known cancer promoter.

The reason why dairy/milk is not healthy is due to the protein in milk. Milk and other dairy products contain casein and have been associated with cancer development. Dr. T. Colin Campbell, in his book, *The China Study*, discovers that casein, which comprises of 85% of the protein in cow's milk, promoted cancer in all stages of its development.

That is why it is recommended that you consider some **milk alternatives**:

Soy Milk

Rice Milk

Almond Milk

Oat Milk

Hemp Milk

Coconut Milk

Type of Milk (1 cup)	Calories	Fat	Sat. Fat	Chol.	Protein	Carbs	Sugars
Whole cow's milk	150	8 g	5 g	35 mg	8 g	12 g	12 g
2% cow's milk	130	5 g	3 g	20 mg	8 g	13 g	12 g
1% cow's milk	110	2.5 g	1.5 g	15 mg	8 g	13 g	12 g
Skim cow's milk	90	0 g	0 g	<5 mg	8g	13 g	12 g
Soy, unsweetened	80-90	4-4.5 g	0.5 g	0 mg	7-9 g	4-5 g	1-2 g
Soy, plain/original	70-130	2-4 g	0-0.5 g	0 mg	5-8 g	8-16 g	6-9 g
Almond, unsweetened	30-50	2.5 g	0 g	0 mg	1 g	1-5 g	0-1 g
Almond, original	50-60	2.5 g	0 g	0 mg	1 g	6-8 g	5-6 g
Hemp, unsweetened	70	6 g	0.5 g	0 mg	2 g	1 g	0 g
Hemp, original	100-140	5-6 g	0.5 g	0 mg	2-4 g	8-20 g	6-14 g
Rice, plain	80-130	2-2.5 g	0 g	0 mg	1 g	16-27 g	8-14 g
Oat, original	110-130	1.5-2.5 g	0 g	0 mg	4 g	24 g	19 g
Hazelnut, original	110	3.5 g	0 g	0 mg	2 g	18 g	14 g
Coconut, unsweetened	50	5 g	5 g	0 mg	1 g	1 g	0 g
Coconut, original	80	5 g	5 g	0 mg	1 g	7 g	6 g

HEALTHY FATS/ GOAL 7: Use the food diary by plugging in how you plan to consume _____ healthy fats this week!

Question 1: How do you **plan** to achieve your healthy fast goal?

Now is a good time to use your food diary. The food diary is going to help you create your personalized meal plan. You may be already consuming foods that are high in fats, the plan is to make the choices appropriate, consistent in servings.

_____

_____

Question 2: How **confident** are you that you can achieve your goal?

How CONFIDENT are you that you will succeed with your plan? (0=not confident; 10=Confident)										
0	1	2	3	4	5	6	7	8	9	10

Question 3: What **obstacles** that may hinder you from achieving your goal?

_____

_____

Question 4: What **strategies** are you going to put in place to help you achieve your goal?

_____

_____

1. Portion Size

Key points: A serving should fit in the palm of your hand

2. Serving size examples

Whole Grain

- 1 slice of whole grain bread

- 4 whole-wheat crackers

- ½ cup of pasta

- 1 cup of ready-to-eat cereal

- 1 whole wheat tortilla (7 inches in diameter)

- ½ cup of couscous

- ½ whole wheat English muffin

Fruit

- 1 medium apple

- 1 handful of strawberries

- 1 small-medium banana

- ¼ cup of dried fruit

- ½ cup of sliced strawberries

- ¼ cup of raisins/dried cranberries

- ¼ of a medium avocado

Vegetables

- 1 cup of raw leafy vegetables

- ½ cup of other vegetables (cooked or raw)

- 3 broccoli florets

- 1 medium sweet potato

- 6 baby carrots (1/2 cup)

- ½ cup of sliced cucumbers

- ½ cup of cherry tomatoes

- ½ cup of tomato sauce

Protein

- 2-3 ounces of cooked meat

- 1 egg

- ½ cup of cooked beans

- 1/3 cup of nuts

Dairy

- 4cubes of cheese (dice size)

- 1 cup of low-fat yogurt (8 oz.)

- 1 cup of low-fat/skim milk (8 oz.)

- ½ cup of cottage cheese

- 1 cup of yogurt

- 1 ½ ounces of cheese